ONE IN TWELVE

Vanessa J E Smith

1997

'Modo liceat vivere, est spes'
'Where there's life, there's hope'
(TERENCE, C. 190-159 B.C.)

Published by The Genesis Appeal 1997,
The Nightingale Centre, South Manchester University Hospitals,
Nell Lane, Manchester M20 0PT

British Library Cataloguing in Publication Data
Smith, Vanessa, 1951 -
One in Twelve
ISBN 0 953087 10 7

Printed in Great Britain by
Dearneside Press, Scissett, Huddersfield, West Yorkshire

DEDICATION

This booklet is dedicated to all those striving to eradicate breast cancer.

FOREWORD

The UK has the highest incidence of breast cancer of anywhere in the world, with over 29,000 women developing the disease each year. Despite many improvements in methods of detecting and treating breast cancer, half will not be cured. For women aged between 35 and 50, breast cancer remains the commonest cause of death. But behind the statistics are real people with real stories to tell - some of heartbreak, some of courage, some of hope. In this book Vanessa Smith has drawn together stories that will make you smile, and stories that will make you cry. All of the profits from this book will go to projects which will improve the early diagnosis and treatment of breast cancer. Your money could not be put to better use.

LESTER BARR (Chairman)

THE GENESIS APPEAL FOR RESEARCH INTO BREAST CANCER

ACKNOWLEDGEMENTS

I would like to thank and acknowledge:

The women (some names changed for confidentiality) who gave up their time to speak to me about such a personal subject;

Everyone at the South Manchester University Hospitals who combined professionalism with care, support and humour, before, during and after my operation, in particular:

Andrew Baildam	Consultant Surgeon
Martin Bellman	Consultant Anaesthetist
Aine Binchy	Genetic Counsellor
Gareth Evans	Consultant Clinical Geneticist
Penny Hopwood	Honorary Consultant Psychiatrist;

My husband Graham, and my children Emmeline and Joshua for providing me with the support and encouragement necessary, not only to undergo a voluntary bilateral mastectomy, but to research and produce this booklet;

COLLAGEN (UK) Ltd., the company which supplied my breast implants, for generously sponsoring this booklet by paying the printing costs;

Pam Glass of the Genesis Appeal for her invaluable help and patience;

Lastly but by no means least, all my friends and relatives who have shared with me the best and the worst moments of the last few years, in particular Wendy for her encouragement throughout and Pat and Ann for being such inspirations.

CONTENTS

INTRODUCTION

by

Vanessa Smith

I was lucky. I did not have breast cancer, but I still had a double mastectomy.

In May 1995, the results of a recently developed genetic test for hereditary breast cancer confirmed that I had inherited a defective gene, BRCA1, from my mother. This gave me an 85-90% probability of developing breast cancer in my lifetime, the disease which had killed my mother and affected eleven out of twelve members of my extended family.

Rather than wait for the cancer to develop, I opted for voluntary bilateral mastectomy, which is a preventative operation in which as much glandular breast tissue as possible is removed from both breasts. The operation took place on January 25th 1996 at the Christie Hospital, Manchester, a Centre of Excellence for the prevention, detection and treatment of cancer. I had immediate reconstruction using Trilucent implants based on vegetable oil, retaining my outer skin and nipples. In just a few hours I had not only reduced my risk of beast cancer from almost certainty to virtually nil, but I had also acquired a wonderful new pair of boobs!

My actions have often been described by others as 'brave' but the genuinely brave women are those who, like the ones in this booklet, have had to face and come to terms with breast cancer. When my mother died in 1984 the word 'cancer' was rarely spoken out loud. It was usually referred to in whispers as 'The Big C'. Few people were willing to talk openly about it. The women in this booklet agreed to speak to me about their experiences, sometimes with humour, sometimes with sadness, in order to show that breast cancer can be faced and successfully fought.

In this country, **ONE IN TWELVE** women develops breast cancer. Genetic research represents the beginning of a cure. It saved me from likely death at an early age. I wish I could say that was the end of the story but I have two young children, Emmeline (aged ten) and Joshua (aged seven), growing up in the knowledge that they, too, may carry the gene.

That is why I am donating all the profits of this booklet to The Genesis Appeal. Thank you for your support.

Vanessa J. E. Smith

A WORD OF ENCOURAGEMENT

by

Diane Modahl, Olympic Athlete

In the summer of 1993, whilst settling down to fall asleep, I discovered a lump in my breast and in the next 48 hours my life changed irretrievably.

My immediate reaction was: "I'm going to die" which, of course, was an irrational reaction but by morning I was more philosophical and clear thinking. I made an appointment with my GP who suggested I see a specialist because "The lump is too big to be ignored" (about the size of a pea).

What made matters worse was that my husband was working away and so I was facing this dilemma alone. The appointment to visit the specialist came through the next day and whilst speaking to my husband on the telephone, he insisted that I didn't go alone. "Why not?" I asked, "I don't want this to become a problem until it is a problem". I won and made him promise not to call my parents and worry them unnecessarily.

So much for the promise! He called my parents and spoke to my father who **did** believe I was going to die and so I found myself consoling him! Nonetheless, I visited the specialist alone and I underwent a biopsy which fortunately turned out to be benign. What a relief.

I visited the specialist for about a year after the initial visit which, thankfully, proved to be a mere precaution and I didn't require any further treatment. Not all of us who experience breast lumps are as fortunate as me and their stories may end quite differently but help and support is available, if not from family and friends, then certainly from the medical profession and support groups.

In my experience as an international runner, athletes do face periods of disappointment and frustration but also happiness and exhilaration when a competition goes according to plan. The same can be said of real life. It is also unpredictable and provides us with challenges, some more difficult than others. However bridges are there to be crossed when we come to them - life is for living and regardless of what adversities are thrown at us we should tackle them as athletes approach their races - with determination, courage and confidence.

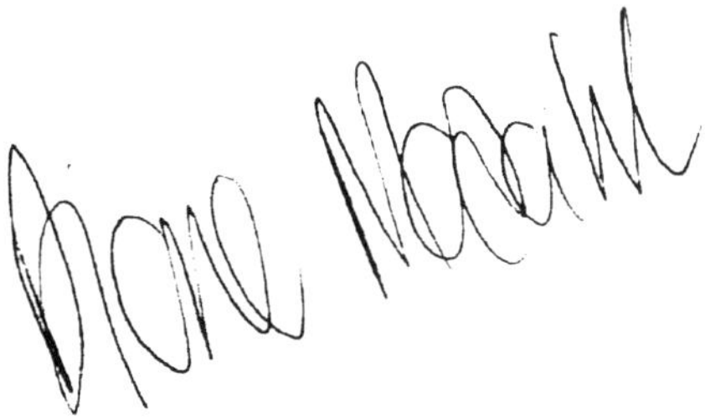

IT REALLY HELPS TO TALK

Lady Mary Ripley discovered she had breast cancer in December 1996, at the age of 63.

Early in December 1996, I went for routine breast screening. My previous mammogram, a year earlier, had shown up what appeared to be abnormal tissue and I had been recalled. I had neglected to mention that I was on HRT and, apparently, it was this which had accounted for the 'abnormality'. The breast tissue had appeared more youthful than it should have done. This time, I remembered to say that I was receiving HRT and so was surprised to be recalled once again. I was not worried, however. If the HRT was not responsible, it would be a benign cyst. My sister had undergone a lumpectomy for two such cysts and this probably ran in the family.

I convinced my husband that he should go to work as normal and I drove to the hospital. There, I had an ultrasound scan and a biopsy. Two hours later, I was in a room with the surgeon and a breast care nurse listening in disbelief as I was told, "I'm sorry but you have some cancerous cells and it does mean surgery."

Suddenly I felt that a huge hole was opening up in front of me. This sort of thing happened to other people, not to me. We have always been very lucky. People looking at us would think we had everything but cancer can happen to anyone. When I was in hospital having my mastectomy, I became very friendly with a cleaner who was also called Mary. One day, I asked her to dispose of some used envelopes for me. Glancing down at them she saw that they were addressed to Lady Ripley. "And I thought you were one of us!" she exclaimed. I had to reassure her that I was indeed "one of us."

I found it easier than I had envisaged to tell people I had breast cancer. I think it was made easier to say the word 'cancer' because the surgeon had said it. He had not disguised my illness by using other words. If this had happened some years ago, I might have found it more difficult because it was not often spoken about openly.

My operation took place on January 2nd, 1997. Just beforehand it felt as though I were heading towards the edge of a precipice. My husband and I used to lie awake at night and weep together. If there is a benefit to having breast cancer it is that the disease brought us closer together. We usually lead such busy lives but we made time to talk more. We have wept together, hugged each other and supported each other. My husband is my reason for getting better.

I have learned to be honest with my feelings. The night before my operation was dreadful. The time passed so slowly. Nurses kept looking in and asking me if I was all right and I always replied that I was. Yet when they had gone, I cried because I was not 'all right'. If they had said "How are you?" I would have found it easier to tell them the truth. After the initial diagnosis, I found myself in the position of consoling others. I was trying to be brave for their sake. There is a certain self-imposed pressure to put on a brave front and to reassure others that one is being positive. I was trying to allay other people's fears and so ignoring my own. Once I admitted to myself and to others just how dreadful I really felt, a weight seemed to be lifted from me. It was not self pity, just honesty. It is important to be allowed to feel 'low' at times.

Two years ago we became involved with the BBC series 'Video Nation Shorts', which intends to preserve a cross-section of society for the BBC archives. These 'shorts' can then be used for future research. When my cancer was diagnosed my husband and I decided to record our feelings. This helped us to be open with each other and made us put feelings into words. What we were having to confront and deal with was so personal and so emotional that I think it would have been hard to be totally honest with each other had we not been involved with this programme.

It is now just over three months since my mastectomy. My husband and I have recently celebrated our Ruby Wedding anniversary and it had an extra special significance for us. We had two reasons to celebrate and we drank plenty of champagne!

I have been given the all-clear and my surgeon says there is no reason why I should not live well into old-age. I am now getting used to my prosthesis, although no-one told me that, initially, I would be unable to wear it all the time. Even now I have to go without it for up to a week as it is heavy and, after a while, becomes uncomfortable. The possibility of reconstructive surgery has been mentioned but I feel it is too soon to think rationally about that. At the moment I cannot bear to think of having more surgery.

It is important to be positive and to be prepared to put up a fight. You must believe that there is a future and, hopefully, I will be around for a long time now!

I LEFT MY LUMP FOR SEVEN YEARS

Annie, now 66 years old, had a mastectomy in 1988, having left a lump in her left breast for seven years.

I never used to examine my breasts. I never even looked at myself in the mirror when undressed until one day and that is when I saw the lump. At the back of my mind I think I knew then what it was but no-one ever talked about 'cancer'. It was a taboo subject. What people referred to as 'The Big C' gave rise to a fear, based on mystery and ignorance. I grew up not bearing even to think about it.

I did not feel ill. On the contrary, I felt particularly well and fit. I had rarely visited the doctor and so I ignored the discovery of my lump and got on with my life. Then, seven years later, the lump started to weep and to stain my bra. That is when I finally decided to visit the doctor. As soon as he saw it, he diagnosed breast cancer. An appointment was made for me to visit the hospital a fortnight later.

In all those seven years I had not mentioned the lump to anyone, not even my husband. When I went to the hospital for my appointment, I went alone, resigned to my fate. I now realised how foolish I had been. My appointment was for a Friday and they wanted to admit me on the Monday but I could not go in so soon. I still had not told my husband or family and I needed time to prepare them. When I told them I had breast cancer they were shocked but they thought I had just discovered the lump! To this day, only the doctors know the truth. My husband and I are a loving couple but we never talk about the cancer.

Whilst I was in hospital I shared a ward with seven other women, all with breast cancer. Six had lumpectomies, myself and another woman had mastectomies. The other lady who had a mastectomy died after three years. One lady, with whom I became quite friendly, discovered another lump three years after her lumpectomy. She had a mastectomy but, two years after that, she was dead. She was only forty-four. I was so shocked. I used to visit her where she worked but on several occasions she was not there. I never asked where she was and I am so very sad about that now; I should have talked to her more.

After my operation I had radiotherapy and chemotherapy. Throughout everything, I just accepted what was happening to me. I never asked any questions. In those days you were brought up to put yourself in the hands of the medics and accept your fate. I thought that, if I died, I had only myself to blame because I had left my lump for so long.

While I was in hospital I reached for something and pulled my arm. I think I broke a stitch then. Back home the wound started to weep. I saw the consultant about it was an out-patient but he just looked at me and said "What do you expect with cancer?". Even the nurse with him looked shocked. He was so uncaring and lacking in sympathy.

I never really had any support after the operation. I have only just been discharged after nine years and to this day no-one has mentioned any support groups. I have problems with bras and would like some advice. I am a thirty-six B, but sometimes the bra is too tight and the prosthesis is uncomfortable and slips. The local high-street stores do not stock mastectomy bras. I think you can get ones with pockets somewhere but I do not know where. In any case, I expect they would be expensive.

No-one has ever mentioned breast reconstruction to me. I think I would like that. I sometimes feel I am not 'whole', not all there. Then I realise it is my fault. If I had gone to the doctor earlier, I might not have had to have a mastectomy, so I must put up with it. I still cry over how stupid I was. I feel so guilty.

Those women who died went to the doctor as soon as they found their lumps. Nine years on, I am still here and I thank God every day for that. I would tell other women not to be like me, not to be frightened. If I found a lump in my other breast, I would go straight to the doctor.

I GAINED A WONDERFUL NEW PAIR AT THE AGE OF FIFTY-SEVEN

In August, 1994, Julie, aged 56, had a voluntary bilateral mastectomy following a long history of cysts in both breasts. One year later, she had reconstructive breast surgery.

For almost twenty-five years, I had suffered from breast-related problems. I had the first cyst when I was thirty-two. Altogether, I had three lumps removed and several aspirations. All of these lumps proved to be benign but in 1991 a routine mammogram and further tests revealed 'carcinoma in situ' in the lobes of both breasts. This meant that I had a 30% probability of developing cancer at some indeterminable time in the future.

My specialist recommended six-monthly mammograms and Tamoxifen. During the following three years, the fear of cancer hung over me like a black cloud. I also worried about the side effects of taking a powerful drug over a long period. Increasingly I disliked the prospect of having my breasts squashed between glass plates every six months for an unknown period of time. Suddenly, it dawned on me that there was an alternative. I was in the enviable position of knowing the score and, moreover, I love life far too much to risk throwing it all away just to keep my breasts intact.

I visited my surgeon and managed to convince him that I was determined to go ahead with what had initially appeared to him a 'radical decision'. My husband fully supported my decision from the very beginning and he was a tower of strength all the way.

The operation was not nearly as traumatic as I had anticipated. In fact, ten days later I had a day out shopping with my daughter and six weeks later I was swimming, playing tennis and generally carrying on with my life as usual. I only told a few close friends because I did not want any fuss, and certainly no sympathy since it was my own decision.

One year later, I had breast reconstruction. I had tissue expander implants, where an 'expander implant' is placed beneath the skin and muscle of the chest and over a period of a few months is gradually filled with saline solution, stretching the skin. The tissue expanders were then replaced with permanent implants. I had the great advantage of being able to decide what size to be! I decided to go for a size slightly larger than my natural breasts and, whereas my breasts had sagged after having three children, these are much firmer. It seemed to me that I just could not lose! In addition, I do not have to undergo regular mammography, I no longer take Tamoxifen and, after twenty-five years, I am without worry of breast cancer.

The only difference my reconstructed breasts have made to me is to make me infinitely more shapely! I can now wear a slinky, strapless dress and a skimpy bikini. On holiday in Paris last year, I decided to treat myself to some expensive French lingerie. As I tried on a particularly sexy bra, the assistant helping me commented, "But Madam, you have such a good bust for your age." If only she knew! At the tennis club I belong to few of the women know of my operation. We are all over forty and most of the women are concerned about their breasts beginning to sag. Only last week, one woman asked how I managed to stay so firm.

I did not keep my nipples because, had I developed cancer, it would most likely have been in the milk ducts. I have artificial ones which stick on and, from a distance, it is impossible to tell that they are not real. They do not come off easily but I am still rather apprehensive when I swim or play tennis. I am now seriously considering nipple reconstruction using my own skin and have an appointment to discuss this with my surgeon.

I would say to anyone who, like me, has a history of breast-related problems, or who knows she is at high risk of breast cancer - do not be afraid; do not wait for it to happen and risk an early death. You can get rid of the problem and take control of your life.

NOW I CAN FLY!

Having breast cancer enabled Emily, aged 67, to overcome her fear, both of water and of flying.

It all started one July morning in 1994. I was standing at the kitchen sink, running the cold water tap, when I felt something damp at the end of my nipple. I thought I had somehow managed to splash myself through my clothes and thought nothing else of it. Several weeks later I felt the same sensation but this time I was not running any water. I had a look and there was what appeared to be a small bubble at the end of my nipple.

I kept calm although I thought that perhaps it was cancer. The following day I went to the doctor. She gave me a thorough examination but could not feel a lump. I had examined my own breasts too and had not felt anything. An appointment was made for me to have a mammogram a few days later. The results shocked me. The discharge was not serious but the mammogram had shown up cancer in my OTHER breast. At first, I was convinced that there had been some mistake but a biopsy showed that I did, indeed, have a cancerous mass in that breast. I was devastated, I just dropped my head and could not say a word.

I had to decide whether to have a full mastectomy with no further treatment or to have a lumpectomy followed by radiotherapy. I discussed it with my family and eventually decided on the mastectomy. The possibility of breast reconstruction was mentioned but, at the time, the only implants on offer were silicone. There had been a great deal of negative publicity about silicone and I was concerned about its safety.

I am reasonably happy with my prosthesis although it does slip at times. One day I found it in the garden! It must have fallen out while I was gardening. I am certainly not afraid to stand in front of a mirror and look at myself. I even undress in public when I go swimming. In fact, I only learned to swim after I had the mastectomy. Until then I had a fear of water. I had never even let water go above my knees. After my operation I decided that if I could beat cancer I could swim. I asked my daughter to teach me and then I went to classes.

I had always been petrified of flying and had never been in a plane. After the mastectomy I thought that, if I could beat breast cancer and my fear of water, I could perhaps overcome my phobia of flying! I could then bring back my own duty-free without relying on others. So, at sixty-five years of age, I found myself at Manchester Airport undergoing a relaxation course for those who are apprehensive about flying. There were 150 of us altogether plus two pilots, cabin crew and psychiatrists. We had an hour's flight and I survived, largely due to the man next to me who let me grab hold of his hand. He was accompanying his wife. She was squeezing his hand tightly on one side and I was grasping his other one. I have now flown to Spain and Malta and am planning my next holiday. I do not think I am quite ready for Australia yet, but who knows?

If I had not had breast cancer, I would not be able to fly or swim. Cancer has changed my life for the better. I eat more healthily now, exercise more and I have also started to attend aromatherapy classes. Beating cancer makes you a stronger person. You acquire a strength from somewhere that helps you through the operation and that strength stays with you. It is important to be positive. When I feel 'down', I look in the mirror, wag a finger at myself and say aloud, "There is nothing wrong with you!" It is also important to talk. Cancer should not be a taboo subject. It should be discussed openly.

DID STRESS CAUSE MY CANCER?

Irene was diagnosed as having breast cancer in 1987 at the age of 59 after a particularly traumatic period in her life. She is convinced that stress played an important part in causing this disease to develop.

I am convinced that stress caused my cancer. In 1987 I went to North America for nine days with my husband, Ted, and a number of business associates. Whilst visiting Niagara Falls at the start of our working holiday, Ted ate a rather greasy cheeseburger. That night he could not stop vomiting and we assumed it was food-poisoning. However, when it continued into the next day and he began showing signs of dehydration whilst travelling by coach to Boston, we decided he should visit the hospital there. After a two hour wait, he was put on a drip to restore the fluid lost and discharged later that day. It was still assumed he had a very severe stomach upset, nothing worse.

Ted's condition continued to deteriorate throughout the next few days and he was becoming very weak. By the last day of our trip, he had lost four stones in weight and it was obvious he would be unable to fly home. By now we were in Washington and he was admitted to the Fairfax Hospital there, where he was given seven enemas and a number of x-rays. The results of the x-rays showed a tumour in his colon. During his subsequent operation there was another shock - he was also full of gall stones. After the operation he looked terrible and I was convinced I would return home a widow. I used to suffer from nerves but I knew I now had to be strong for Ted's sake. I was in a foreign country and was faced with the prospect of Ted dying but I found strength from somewhere. We were in Washington for seven weeks and I did not allow myself to cry until we arrived home with Ted well on the way to recovery.

A little while after returning home I received an appointment for my regular mammogram. A few days after my appointment I was shocked to receive a note saying I should consult a specialist as the mammogram had revealed a shadow on one breast. A needle biopsy subsequently showed that, what I had prayed would be a benign cyst, was in fact something more sinister.

I was advised to have a mastectomy and, from the beginning, I was determined to be positive and fight this thing. I think attitude is very important in overcoming any illness.

The day I came out of hospital I was told my father had died that morning. He had been very ill for a number of years and I had been spending an increasing amount of time caring for him which, in itself, had been very stressful.

I asked my surgeon if he thought stress had caused my cancer. He could not say for certain but, in my own mind, I am sure that was the cause. I had been coping with looking after my father and then had to cope with being in America for seven weeks with Ted seriously ill. Now I just get on with my life and, in fact, I worked until I was 65. Of course, I have had 'down' moments but Ted and I are very close. We have always been able to talk about our illnesses and we have always been there for each other.

WE HAVE A FAMILY HISTORY OF BREAST CANCER

Jennifer was 32 years old when her cancer was first diagnosed. As a result of the family history of breast cancer, her 23 year old daughter was offered a genetic test. The result was positive.

I was only 32 years old when I discovered I had breast cancer. It was on the day that Prince Charles married Diana, in 1981. I was on a caravanning holiday in Cornwall with my husband and two small children. We had spent most of the day watching the wedding on television and when I was in bed that evening I stretched out and suddenly felt a lump the size of an egg. When I put my arm down, it seemed to disappear.

I was not particularly worried by the lump but decided to visit my own doctor on returning home. He reassuringly told me it was nothing more than a 'breast mouse' which meant that the lump moved freely, an indication that it was a benign cyst. No further appointments were made, so I went home and forgot about it for several months until I had to visit the doctor for an unrelated problem. This time, it was not my own doctor and to this day I do not know why I did it, but as I was leaving the room I turned and heard myself saying, "Could you just look at this lump? I am a little worried as my sister died of cancer last year." My sister had not died of breast cancer but something must have been in my subconscious. The doctor examined me and commented that he was in agreement with the diagnosis made by my own GP, but that he would make a hospital appointment for me in order to be certain. A week later I found myself in hospital having the lump removed.

Soon after being discharged from hospital, I received a letter asking me to return. Unconcerned, I went alone by car. There, the surgeon told me that tests had revealed my lump to be 'a nasty one' and that I would need to have 'the big operation'. I guessed he meant a mastectomy but even the surgeon could not say the words 'cancer' or 'mastectomy'. Back home, I burst into tears and told my husband that I thought I had cancer and needed to have the breast removed although no-one had actually said so. Fortunately, the cancer must have been caught in its early stages and I did not require any further treatment after the operation.

I think I coped better because I was so young. Not once did I think I might die. It never occurred to me that death could be an option. My husband had always been the one to go out to work and I had remained at home with the children, so coping whilst I was in hospital proved difficult for him. The day the children visited me and announced they had been given ravioli on toast for breakfast decided it - I had to get well, and quickly!

Seven years later I discovered another lump in my remaining breast, this time in a different place and more of a thickening than a distinct lump. The results of a biopsy indicated that there was nothing to worry about so, once again, I went into hospital for a lumpectomy. However, the day I was due to leave hospital, I was informed that subsequent tests had revealed the lump to be malignant. I would have to remain in hospital and have a mastectomy.

In many ways, this second mastectomy did not cause me concern. I had lived though the first diagnosis of cancer and, in fact, I had often complained that having just one breast was a nuisance. It seemed to get in the way! Having both breasts removed actually made things easier.

Several years after my second mastectomy, my mother was diagnosed with breast cancer. She was in her early 70's and because of her age was advised to have a lumpectomy. However, it spread to her liver and that is what killed her. My maternal aunt developed breast cancer when I was only eight but she lived until she was 83 years old.

As a result of our family history of breast cancer my daughter Helen, who is now 23, has received genetic counselling. Two years ago she decided to have the newly developed genetic test and, as we had all expected, the result was positive. This means she has an 85-90% probability of developing breast cancer. None of us were surprised at the result; in fact, had it been negative, we just would not have believed it.

We feel that breast cancer does not have to be a death sentence. My mother and aunt lived until old-age and my aunt, in particular, survived many years after cancer had been diagnosed. I have had breast cancer twice but I am very much alive! I have been asked several times if I would have had children had I known I could pass on this gene. Of course I would! You cannot put your life on hold because of the threat of cancer; that would be surrendering to the disease.

My daughter will be monitored regularly once she gets into her late 20's. Whether or not she will eventually have a voluntary mastectomy depends on what alternatives will be available to her. Like me she is very positive. The word 'cancer' has never been a taboo subject in our house and we are not afraid of it.

My lack of breasts has only troubled me when I have been swimming. I have visions of one of the prostheses floating away. It has never bothered my husband either. Bits of me may have been taken away but there are plenty of other bits left!

MY RETIREMENT PRESENT WAS BREAST CANCER

Margaret was diagnosed as having breast cancer two weeks after she retired.

I retired from working as a physiotherapist at the end of August 1986. My leaving party marked (or so I thought) the end of my hospital life. How wrong I was! Just over two weeks later, I accidentally discovered a small lump in my left breast whilst showering. Although I had worked in hospitals for much of my life, I had not seriously considered breast cancer. I never self-examined my breasts and there were no routine mammograms in those days for women over 50 years old. I was invited for cervical smears but not mammography.

Prior to discovering the lump I had no symptoms whatsoever. Convinced it would be nothing serious, I delayed seeing a doctor for a couple of weeks. Within ten days of that appointment I was in hospital undergoing a lumpectomy. I later had radiotherapy which gave me tremendous pain in my shoulder joints and in the muscles of my back. Apparently, I had a very abnormal muscle reaction.

The previous year one of my daughters, who was in her late 20's, had become very ill. She underwent a repair operation on her oesophagus. She appeared to make a good recovery but the day after she was discharged from hospital she suffered severe chest pains and was readmitted with a pulmonary embolism. I took unpaid leave for three months and was at her bedside daily. My daughter recovered but I had suffered enormous stress. I am certain it was no coincidence that one year later I developed breast cancer.

Two years after my operation, during a routine appointment with my consultant, I happened to mention that I felt I was rather lop-sided. I have quite large breasts but the lumpectomy had resulted in a whole bra cup-size difference between breasts. I was only being frivolous when I mentioned this but my consultant asked me if I would like to see a plastic surgeon. Ten months later, surgery reduced the size of my healthy breast and I was the proud owner of a perfectly symmetrical pair!

Almost immediately after my lumpectomy I signed on at University as a mature student of Philosophy. My subsequent success in gaining a degree went to my head and I followed it with a Masters Degree in Health Ethics. I am now learning to slow down and am enjoying my eight grandchildren, walking and playing bridge. Looking back, discovering my lump and having the lumpectomy was little more than a hiccup in my life. Breast cancer does not have to kill. It is possible to overcome it and to go on to live a quality life.

MY MASTECTOMY: A POEM

The author of this poem, who wishes to remain anonymous, has a family history of cancer. She, herself, has been treated for lumps in the breast on numerous occasions over the past five years. Recently, there had been evidence of cells changing and becoming cancerous. Having been warned that she could develop breast cancer at any time in the future, she chose to have a voluntary double mastectomy and wrote this poem whilst in hospital.

MY MASTECTOMY

I'm sitting here in my hospital bed
surrounded by flowers and cards;
some say 'good luck', some 'all the best'
and some offer kindest regards.

I've been in the bath, put on my gown
"Now please don't use talcum", they said
My temperature's taken, I've been robbed of blood
and told I must stay in bed.

I glance around my neighbouring patients;
they're sitting in gowns just like me,
tapping their fingers or dozing
and dying for that cup of tea.

The nurses are hustling and bustling;
they've always got something to do,
a patient is pressing the buzzer
she's wanting to go to the loo.

A nurse seems to pop up from nowhere,
says, “Yes”, she can go for a wee;
with her gown at the back flying open
she’s off, and her bum we all see.

I’m now lying back on my pillow
thinking of what is to come,
waiting for my turn to theatre
wishing my op had been done.

After months of confusion and worry
with the threat of cancer in view,
I want to get this ordeal over
and start to think positive too.

Then quick as a flash I am jolted
out of my day-dreaming state;
“Are you Mrs Jones?” asks the porter
“I am”, I reply, “I can’t wait.”

With the help of a couple of nurses
the trolley I’m lifted upon;
my gown is now round my waistline
my dignity’s got up and gone!

At last I am laid on the trolley,
a paper cap placed on my head;
my modesty’s now under the blankets,
I pray they won’t bring me back dead.

The porter is cheerful and chatty.
"Outside it is lovely" says he
but the weather's not my concern now
for the theatre sign I can see.

He wheels me up to the doorway;
to God I say a quick prayer,
the surgeon is scrubbed up and waiting
I now must go into his lair.

The anaesthetist gives me the needle,
at last I am having my op.
I'm drifting off into dreamland
my boobs are now getting the chop!

I wake up a few hours later
flat chested, thoughts hazy and dim.
What have they done with my boobies?
I bet they've been thrown in the bin!

I'm looking down at my chest now,
it's padded, there's nothing to see.
I convince myself I'm still female
just minus my thirty four B.

A few days from now I'll be wearing
prostheses tucked into my bra,
hoping they'll stay where I put them
and looking quite real from afar.

Soon I will have reconstruction
with boobs that are filled up with gel,
hoping I'll look like a model,
knowing that no-one can tell.

So, if you are having mastectomy,
don't be filled with despair;
your worry of cancer is over
and think of that shapely new pair!

Anon

NOT THE "GOOD OLD DAYS"

Nora is now 78 and had her mastectomy twenty-five years ago.

The cruellest part of having cancer is the way it creeps up on you so silently. When I found my lump, I had not felt ill or experienced any pain. I had just been feeling a little more tired than usual.

I never self-examined my breasts. It was twenty-five years ago and you just did not touch your own breasts in those days. One night, I accidentally touched my breast and felt a small lump. Quietly, without disturbing my husband, I made a cup of tea. Hesitantly, I felt my breast again and the lump was still there. I could still feel it in the morning so, without mentioning it to my husband, I made a doctor's appointment. He referred me to the hospital and ten days later I went in for a needle biopsy. My husband now knew and came with me. His support helped me immensely.

A week later I returned to the hospital to have the stitches out. The surgeon I saw then was not the one who had performed the biopsy. Scrutinising my breast, which was black and blue with bruises, he remarked, "Well, they did a good job of your breast when they did the biopsy, but we have found cancer." It was so abrupt: no sympathy. I was distraught. He proceeded to tell me that I needed a mastectomy, but that he could not do it for over two weeks as it was Easter and he was on holiday. He did, however, suggest his Registrar could do it: "He only has one more exam to do and he will be fully qualified." Once again, I was both shocked and distressed. I have never forgotten that. I refused to even consider his suggestion and left the hospital in tears.

Back home, I just wept. I sat down and smoked non-stop. I must have looked dreadful because my husband said, "You don't look at all well. Are you smoking too much?" Smoking too much! I had virtually eaten cigarettes all day! I heeded those words, though. I put out my cigarette and have not smoked since. So I suppose if I had not had breast cancer, I might have died of lung cancer.

I was still distressed. In those days it was always thought that, if you had cancer, you would automatically die. I was also concerned about who would carry out my operation. A few days later I bumped into a friend who was a physiotherapist at the hospital and she gave me the name of another surgeon. As it happened, he was the one who had performed my biopsy. I contacted him and he agreed to operate on Easter Monday. There were only four of us on the ward because it was during the holidays and my treatment was first-class.

When I left hospital I needed to have a prosthesis fitted. I had to go to the manufacturer's to buy it and, to my horror, the 'falsie' was fitted by a man! He was nothing to do with the medical profession and there was no nurse present, just him and me. I felt so degraded. It nearly finished me off. I could never have gone back. As it happened I could never wear it because it was so very uncomfortable. It had the texture of a beanbag.

Things are different now; the prostheses are fitted at the hospital. When I was discharged I was not offered any advice or given any help. A breast care nurse visited me at home but, when I remarked how lucky I was that all the cancer had been removed, her only words were "Oh, you can't guarantee that, you know - it spreads." I will never forget those words. It was such a cruel thing to say.

My husband was a tower of strength throughout my ordeal. He was very supportive. The cancer was obviously caught in its early stages. I regularly examine my other breast now. I know how crucial it is to self-examine your breasts and go straight to the doctor with a lump.

WILL BREAST CANCER HEAL MY MARRIAGE?

Jocelyn was diagnosed with breast cancer in May 1995 at the age of 42 and after the break-up of her marriage.

Early in 1995, I first noticed that the nipple on my right breast had become inverted. I also had pain in this breast. At first I did not pay too much attention and thought that, since I was 42 years old, it might be due to hormonal changes in my body. I assumed that one day it would return to normal. A few months later, however, I noticed that my breast was changing colour and becoming darker. I had been shown how to examine my breasts by my local doctor but I did not do so regularly. I had very lumpy breasts anyway and thought I would not know which lump should be there and which should not. Just before I noticed these changes in my breast, my marriage had virtually broken down. I had left home and was feeling very stressed so I was not really looking after myself. My thoughts were on the state of my marriage, not of my breasts.

Soon after noticing the discolouring I went away on holiday. There, my attitude changed dramatically from not taking much notice of the changes to becoming panic-stricken, so much so that I visited a doctor there. He tried to calm my fears and said it could be anything but that I should visit my own doctor when I returned home. When I did see my own doctor a fortnight later, he was very concerned as he felt a lump and he advised me to see a specialist. Five weeks later I had a mastectomy, followed by chemotherapy and radiotherapy.

I think the worst problem of all for me was one of ignorance. Beforehand, I knew virtually nothing about breast cancer. I did not even know the incidence of it for women in my age group. Now I know that not having children put me at a higher risk. I have also read that stress is a possible trigger and, if that is so, my personal circumstances at the time would have made me a prime candidate.

My faith as a born-again Christian helped me cope with the ordeal. I was never afraid of dying, but I worried about the likely pain level. I trusted (and still do) that God was in charge no matter what happened and that He would help me through it. This did not insure me against the trauma of chemotherapy, however - I was very sick for the five months I received treatment and I suffered dreadfully.

I also found that it helped enormously to talk to other women who had undergone similar experiences but it is important only to listen to to those who are positive. Talking to others helped allay my fears and made me optimistic that I could go through with the operation and treatment and that I would come out the other side ready to go forward. I am now virtually back to full health and am considering breast reconstruction. I have an appointment to see a plastic surgeon as I believe that reconstruction will help me feel 'whole' again.

Throughout my illness, my husband stood by me. I moved back in with him and, together, we have had to learn to be calmer and to put our marital problems aside. This was a much more immediate battle that needed fighting. It would be naive to believe that breast cancer has rescued our marriage. We still have a very long way to go but we are now pulling together for the first time in a number of years.

I still do not examine my remaining breast. I know some women will find that strange but it is my way of coping. I want to believe that my problems are all over and that I am now free of cancer. I do not want to go searching for it. If a problem does arise, then I will face it when it happens but, for now, I want to forget my ordeal and just get on with my life.

If anyone facing breast cancer would like to talk to me, I am very willing to be contacted through Genesis.

LUMPECTOMY OR MASTECTOMY

Diane developed breast cancer two years ago at the age of 45. She had then to decide between a lumpectomy or a mastectomy.

I occasionally examined my own breasts but, more often than not, I was too busy to take the time. One night in 1995, I turned over in bed and my hand brushed my breast. It was then that I felt a very small lump, no larger than a pea. It was underneath my breast and I always imagined cancer to start on the top, so I did not worry at first. The following morning I mentioned it to my husband and he persuaded me to see a doctor. If I had not gone to the doctor immediately I think I would have left the lump for a while to see if it grew.

After my doctor had examined me, I knew it was serious. The words were reassuring but the tone of the voice had changed. Three days later I had a needle biopsy and a mammogram. The mammogram showed up a dark area much larger than I had envisaged. My husband was devastated and I became breathless and panic-stricken. When I told my parents, who live close by, they were very distressed and we all had a good cry.

After that, my attitude became far more positive. I told my children (aged eighteen and twenty) that I had a growth which needed removing. I could not use the word 'cancer'; I thought that would be too frightening for them, but they guessed.

I had to make the decision whether to have a lumpectomy or a mastectomy. If I had a lumpectomy I would require a course of radiotherapy, but if I opted for a mastectomy no further treatment would be necessary. What a decision to have to make! I am very small-breasted and thought that a mastectomy would not make much difference. However, whilst some of the nurses supported my decision, my friends were horrified at the idea. In the end I asked my surgeon to decide and he chose the lumpectomy.

Three days before I was due to go into hospital I fell heavily whilst running up the garden steps. I hit my leg on a stone slab and it swelled up dreadfully. I thus found myself in casualty. When I went in to have the lumpectomy three days later the operation nearly had to be delayed because I had a temperature and a slight infection in my leg. Fortunately, a course of antibiotics soon brought my temperature down and my operation went ahead as planned.

The day after the operation I was wheeled down to the X-Ray Department so my leg could be x-rayed. I felt such a terrible mess. My hair was greasy, I felt dreadfully sick after the anaesthetic and I thought everyone was looking at me. I was left in the X-Ray Department for almost an hour as there was no-one available to take me back to the ward. When I did arrive back, totally exhausted and still feeling very nauseous, I was met by an army of visitors. I just could not cope. I did not want to see anyone except for my husband. I felt so ill and miserable. It was a relief to leave hospital. It is wonderful to have support but at times that support can be overwhelming. Visiting should be restricted. It was open visiting, all day long, but immediately after my operation I did not really want to see so many people all at once.

Whilst I was in hospital I visited the bathroom, only to find someone else in my bed when I returned! Lack of funds had meant that the ward had to double as a clinic and the lady in my bed was receiving chemotherapy. It was all very hygienic, with clean covers on the bed but it was still my bed! I had to wait in the Day Room until they had finished.

It was suggested to me that I might have reconstructive surgery but, at the time, I felt I had gone through enough and that, after all, I had not had a mastectomy. I am embarrassed and self-conscious about my shape, however. I still play squash but I have stopped going to the gym at my local leisure club. It is full of 'beautiful people' and I am certain that they would notice. When I wash, I wash less vigorously down that side. It does not hurt; I just do not like to touch it. It never bothers my husband but it bothers me.

I feel a great deal of anger because my surgeon suggested that my taking the contraceptive pill over a long period could have increased my risk of breast cancer. I started taking it as a student and, in those days, it was high in oestrogen. I just had no idea that it could be harming me.

My anger has been channelled in a positive direction. It has made me push myself harder and made me determined to beat breast cancer. I have managed to fight it, but I cannot bring myself to visit anyone worse off than me. It might sound selfish but I do not want a constant reminder of what happened to me. I just want to try to forget it.

HAVING BREAST CANCER LED TO A NEW INTEREST

Cath Davies, aged 52, is the Founder of the Sheffield Breast Cancer Care Group.

I was forty-nine when, in February 1993, breast cancer was diagnosed. I never used to examine my own breasts; cancer was never at the forefront of my mind. Then, one day whilst in the bath, I noticed an inverted nipple. I called my husband and told him, "I think WE have a problem!"

The following day, by coincidence, I had a doctor's appointment for a completely unrelated matter. When the doctor examined my breast he agreed that there did seem to be a problem. That was February 18th and, when my appointment came through to see a consultant, it was for the end of March. I had not realised I would have to wait so long. It was then that I remembered I had private health insurance. I rang the doctor and suggested I go privately. Two days later I got an appointment! Cancer was diagnosed and a bed reserved for me for the very next afternoon. Everything happened so quickly that I never really had time to worry. In fact, the following morning I went into work. I am responsible for the salaries and I wanted to make sure I got paid!

I had a mastectomy and my lymph glands removed and one month later returned to work on a part-time basis. That was when my life took another unexpected dramatic turn. I was approached by a colleague and asked if I would speak to another lady who worked there. This lady had undergone a mastectomy a year before and was still very depressed. So, just five weeks after my own operation, I found myself trying to comfort someone else. I was shocked to discover how little she knew compared to me. She was taking Tamoxifen, but did not know why. Nothing had been explained to her. The prosthesis kept slipping and showing above her overalls but she knew nothing about mastectomy bras with pockets.

I decided to ring my hospital to get the name of a support group and I was once again shocked to discover there was not one. When I mentioned this to my surgeon he asked if I would like to set one up.

I tentatively suggested the idea to my husband and this time it was his turn to be shocked. After all, it was still only a few weeks after my mastectomy. However, we agreed that I should give it a try and, in October 1993, the Sheffield Breast Care Group was founded.

Gradually, I began to realise that the lady at work was not alone in her ignorance. As a private patient I appeared to have been the privileged recipient of information not imparted to NHS patients. I was also to discover that their quality of care was less than mine. My surgeon was very understanding. He gave me his home telephone number and told me to ring him at any time. This caring manner really helped me but I know that NHS patients are treated differently.

I was determined that all women should have equal access to information. The Group now has regular meetings, drop-ins and a club for young women with breast cancer. We also do home visits and the telephone line is always open.

We produce many leaflets about all aspects of breast cancer and these are available free of charge. We now have 247 members, including some who have had a positive result to a genetic test. We have also had a man with breast cancer. Often, coming home after the operation is when people feel at their lowest and most vulnerable. They are so well looked after in hospital that they feel isolated when discharged. As one women said, it is like suddenly coming to the end of a conveyor belt. That is when they most need to talk to someone.

Forming this support group has helped me enormously. It has kept me going and kept me positive. I could not have done it without my husband's support although one day he jokingly asked if he could make an appointment to see me. At the time I laughed but then I thought that perhaps he was coming second. I suggested to him that I should give up and let someone else take over the group. "Of course not!" he replied emphatically, "There are too many people out there needing help."

Exactly one year after my mastectomy I had breast reconstruction. Although I was a private patient it had not been suggested. I had to ask for it. Years before, I had read an article about breast reconstruction and had remembered it. I have also had a nipple made, although not from my own skin. It was colour-coded to match the other one and it is difficult to tell which is the real one.

Cancer definitely changes your attitude to things. For my husband, it was probably most difficult for him to come to terms with the transformation in my personality rather than the difference in my physical appearance. I now question everything - something which I did not do before. The physical change was never a problem. Neither of us ever believed it would be.

IT WAS NOT HAPPENING TO ME

Betty was fifty-six when she found a lump in 1994. She coped with her cancer by pretending it was not happening to her.

I never used to think about breast cancer. In our family there is a history of heart problems but I only know of two aunts on my father's side who have suffered from breast cancer. I had thought about the possibility of dying from a heart attack but never from cancer.

When breast cancer was diagnosed, it was such a shock. It just could not be happening to me! It all started one night, three years ago, just six months after my annual mammogram. I adjusted my bra strap and suddenly felt a lump under my arm the size of a plum! As it happened, I had a doctor's appointment a couple of days later for something different and my daughter insisted I mention the lump then. When I did, the doctor's face dropped but I would not believe it could be cancer. Even when, a few days later, I found myself in hospital having a needle biopsy, it was not happening to me. It was someone else lying there. I could not possibly have breast cancer; heart disease, yes, but not cancer.

When the consultant confirmed the diagnosis, I was speechless, but I still refused to believe it. As I left the hospital I bumped into a friend who enquired about my health. "I'm fine, except they have just told me I've got breast cancer," I replied! Everyone else was upset but not me. My husband burst into tears. He drinks and smokes and said it was unfair that I had never abused my body yet had cancer. I never thought like that, though, because it was not happening to me. It never occurred to me that I might die; in fact it was all a big inconvenience. I suppose that was my way of coping.

After the needle biopsy, it took two weeks to get the results. Three days later I had the lump removed. However, when I went back to the clinic, I was told I would have to go into hospital again as I still had some cancerous cells and this time I would need to have my lymph glands removed. Following this operation, I had radiotherapy and then chemotherapy. The first dose of chemotherapy made me dreadfully ill. In five days I lost 9lbs but I had read articles about how terrible chemotherapy is and I thought I must just put up with it. All I could do was lie down. Friends and family urged me to go to the doctor but I just accepted it. When I eventually told them at the hospital, they were furious with me. They changed all my medication and kept me in whilst I underwent my second treatment. I was not nearly so ill; just very tired, You are told chemotherapy can make you ill but not how ill is **TOO** ill.

The medical staff who looked after me were fantastic, especially Valerie, my breast care nurse. It was like being a private patient. All my questions were answered fully and sympathetically. As time went on, however, I began to feel that I was losing control of my life. It had been taken over by medics. I was totally in their hands. Then, suddenly, the unexpected happened. Once all the treatment had finished and I was given back control of my own life, I could not cope. I felt a gap in my life and, for the first time since cancer was diagnosed, I started to worry. Words like 'cancer', 'radiotherapy' and 'chemotherapy' now frightened me.

The thought of cancer started to consume me. Anyone who asked how I was now got the whole lot, from thread to needle. No longer did I reply breezily "I'm fine, thank you." I talked to, and bored everyone. Every Thursday night for a long time I said a prayer for all the women who were going to clinic the following day. I became obsessional. I would go into a newsagents and scan the covers of magazines for articles on breast cancer. If there was anything about it on television I would make sure I watched it. I felt part of a private club. I just could not let go.

After six months of this my daughter, in desperation, rang Valerie and asked her to visit me. When Valerie arrived and asked what was worrying me, I replied that nothing was. I thought I was behaving quite rationally! However, I did ask Valerie if she thought the cancer would return. I will never forget her reply: "Well, supposing it does, Betty? If it does and you're worrying now, you will have wasted valuable time, and if it doesn't, it will be the same." Those were the most meaningful words anyone had spoken.

It is now three years since I found my lump. I am no longer consumed with the thought of cancer. I occasionally read articles about it, but I also get on with my life. The other night I picked up a magazine to read in bed. There was an article about finding lumps and I just skipped those pages.

I will never forget what happened to me and sometimes I do feel 'down'. I never take my health for granted now. Sometimes, when I am really enjoying myself, I have a sudden feeling that something will happen to take the enjoyment away. Cancer does change you; I never used to feel like that.

When I first saw my surgeon, I mentioned that two paternal aunts had suffered from breast cancer and asked if it could be hereditary. At the time, I was told that breast cancer could not have been passed on through my father, only my mother. Now genetic research shows that is not the case, so my cancer may have been hereditary.

The possibility of breast reconstruction was mentioned to me but I did not have a mastectomy and the scar is underneath my arm and hardly noticeable. I always self-examine my breasts now. It is something that all women should do.

LIFE CAN STILL BE WONDERFUL AFTER MASTECTOMIES

Elizabeth discovered new happiness at the age of 64, after two mastectomies and the tragic loss of her first husband.

In 1971, at the age of 45, I discovered a lump in my left breast. At that time I never self-examined my breasts and found it quite accidentally whilst showering. After a biopsy, I was referred to a specialist who advised me that I needed an operation. If, during the operation, tests showed the lump to be cancerous, the breast would be removed, otherwise I would have a lumpectomy.

Immediately prior to the operation and on the advice of my surgeon, I went away on a holiday which had been arranged for some time. I returned feeling relaxed and healthy. In fact, I had always felt fit. I used to swim and horse-ride regularly and always looked after myself. I was thus convinced that the lump must be benign and I went into hospital feeling extremely positive.

Immediately after the operation I looked down at my chest. I could see lots of bandages but there was no breast. I was devastated. Although the possibility of losing a breast had been mentioned, neither my husband nor myself had prepared ourselves. I just had not been able to envisage losing a part of my body when I felt so well. I received no counselling and I came out of hospital with cotton wool tucked inside my bra. I fastened my prosthesis to my bra with ribbon but, when I bent down it fell out. I knew nothing of mastectomy bras until I saw an advert for them in Lady magazine. I wish reconstructive surgery had been available then as I would have appreciated that.

After the mastectomy I began self-examining my remaining breast and, four years later, I discovered a lump in that breast. The surgeon recommended a mastectomy and this time I was more prepared as I knew beforehand what was going to happen to me. I also had my lymph glands removed and so was in much more pain than previously. Within an hour of being discharged from hospital there was a knock at my door and there was a policeman standing on the doorstep. My husband had gone into work and collapsed with a massive heart attack. One hour later, I was by his bedside in the Intensive Care Unit. He was only in his early fifties and there had been no history of heart problems. Fortunately, he survived. It seemed that stress had caused it. After my first mastectomy the surgeon had informed my husband that my lump had been malignant but, because I was in such a state of shock, my husband was advised to tell me it had been benign. The second lump was also malignant but, again, my husband kept the truth from me. He only told me just before he died, nine years after the first heart attack. In spite of the fact that I had undergone two mastectomies, I was more than happy to believe this. I never questioned it.

My husband, however, had to live with the stress of knowing the truth but, at the same time, keeping it from me. In 1984, nine years after my husband's first heart attack, I came home from work to find him upstairs lying on the bed feeling unwell. An hour later he was dead. He had suffered another major heart attack.

I was alone for the next four years and then, whilst staying with a friend in another part of the country, I met Tom, a widower. We hit it off immediately. We had similar personalities, we were both active and outgoing and we enjoyed the same things. Over the next few years we travelled up and down the country visiting each other and in 1989, at the age of 64, I remarried. I had mentioned my mastectomies very soon after meeting Tom for the first time and it has never made any difference to our relationship.

We now live life to the full. When I married I immediately acquired six grandchildren. We travel all over Britain and the world and we are constantly planning something new. Life really is wonderful. My story shows that, even late on in life and after two mastectomies, it is possible to fall in love and build a new fulfilling life.

TO FIGHT OR NOT TO FIGHT

In 1991, Frances discovered she had breast cancer. Five years later her husband died of prostate cancer.

I discovered my lump in July 1991 at the age of 65. I was taking a shower at the end of a particularly warm and beautiful summer's day when I felt a slight swelling in my right breast. There was no pain, even when I touched it, and it was not visible when I looked at myself in the mirror. I assumed I must have knocked it whilst playing with my grandchildren. I gave it a quick rub and forgot about it until two weeks later when I felt it again. It had not grown; it was still not painful; it would be nothing serious. However, I did decide to mention it to my doctor although I felt certain I would be wasting his time. Ten days later, I was in hospital having a biopsy and lumpectomy.

The results of the biopsy were due two weeks later. During that time I learned to cope with the '4.00am Will..ies': Will it be malignant? Will I have to go back to hospital? Will it be painful? Will I die?

When I eventually returned to the hospital for the results, the specialist did not waste words but told me in as kindly a manner as possible: "The results are positive. You have breast cancer." What horrors those two words 'breast cancer' conjure up! All my worst fears were encapsulated in those two short words. How would I cope? I had no pre-prepared strategy; cancer had never been part of my life.

After the initial shock, I sat down and tried to think logically. It was then that I realised just how much fear was contained within the word 'cancer' itself. Did I really believe it was going to kill me? After much deliberation I decided that, if it was, it would not be without a fight. Life was too precious just to throw away. When I told my family, I made a conscious effort to say the word 'cancer'. It did not come easily; it is a hard word to say because of the many emotions attached to it.

The reaction of other people was that I could not possibly have it. I was too fit, too well and I had too much energy. However, cancer is not a respector of persons. It hits both the fit and the not-so-fit.

One night, in my mind, I wrote two columns: reasons to live and reasons not to live. The former column was by far the longer. That decided it: I would fight this thing!

Ten days after the diagnosis I went into hospital for a mastectomy. Most of the time prior to the operation I was on a high because of all the support I received. When I did feel low, I prayed. I have always believed in the power of prayer. Immediately after the operation I knew it would not be the end of my life. My life would be different but it would still be good. I looked at my body straight away. It has never been beautiful. All my life I have been a little plump lady. Now, all I could think was how neat the scar was. The surgeon had done a wonderful job. Reconstructive surgery was mentioned but I felt the money could be put to better use elsewhere. The NHS does not have so much money and, although my husband and I were very loving, he was not well and our sex life was over.

My husband Philip, had suffered from a heart condition for many years and, two years after my operation, he had a stroke. He made an almost full recovery from that but, in June 1996, fate dealt us another bitter blow and he was diagnosed as having prostate cancer. From that moment he seemed to lose heart. He became more and more sedentary, which was totally out of character. He stopped eating and gradually he lost both weight and strength. Yet his treatment for cancer appeared to be working.

If I tried to make him laugh he would tell me not to be so cheerful. Looking back, I feel that once Philip's cancer had been diagnosed, he gave up hope of there being any more good life. When he talked he always said that he did not want life without quality and, as far as he was concerned, there could be no quality of life after cancer.

I had to choose my words very carefully. I once said, "But Philip, lots of people have cancer and get better." Philip interpreted that as my saying that I had overcome cancer, so why could he not do the same? It was not what I had meant but it made me realise that everyone must deal with cancer in their own way. I also believe that, to overcome it, you must be prepared to fight it. At the end Philip went into a hospice. He was very peaceful there and he died with dignity.

It was what he wanted. Whether his way of dealing with cancer was right or wrong or whether my way was right or wrong, we each got what we had wished for. Cancer has taken away from me the husband who shared my life for over half a century but, so far, my own fight has been won.

Tomorrow is the first day of the rest of my life.

I CLIMBED DOWN THE WALL OF THE HOSPITAL

Pamela's mastectomy, at the age of 52, opened up a host of new opportunities, including the chance to abseil down her hospital wall.

I've only got one
But then some have got none
Then there's those who've got two
Who cry, "What shall I do?"

They're too big
They're too small
They sag to the right
They sag to the left,"

Just be thankful
Be careful
Look after your breasts

Pamela

I never thought cancer could happen to me, only to other people. I was very fit. I did not smoke, I swam 30 lengths three times a week, I cycled six miles to work every day and I ate a healthy diet.

I was receiving HRT treatment and, as part of my six-monthly check-ups, my doctor always examined my breasts. So why me? My battle (for that was what it was) with breast cancer began in 1992 when I accidentally discovered a lump underneath my right arm. I went to the doctor's the same day. My General Practitioner was on holiday and the doctor I saw thought it was nothing to worry about but said she would make me a hospital appointment.

It was 13 unforgettable weeks between finding the lump and having my mastectomy. During those 13 weeks a mammogram showed up another lump, this time in the breast itself. I had two biopsies from each lump as, on both occasions, the first biopsy was inconclusive.

All this time I felt no physical pain; I just felt confused and very helpless. I could not sleep because I was conscious of this 'thing' growing inside me. I read everything I could find on breast cancer but it would have helped to have spoken to another woman who had gone through the same thing. The waiting period was the most stressful part and, at times, it was almost unbearable for both myself and my husband.

The day I went into hospital a nurse brought me the consent form to sign. I always read everything carefully before signing and seeing the word 'mastectomy' with the letter 'L' next to it, I asked what the 'L' stood for. I prayed it did not mean that the surgeon was a Learner, but I was equally shocked by the nurse's reply:
"It means Left," she said.
"Left what?" I asked innocently.
"Left breast, of course."
For a moment I was speechless then somehow I managed to find sufficient voice to utter, "But it's my right breast that has the cancer!"

Immediately, the nurse corrected the mistake on the paper and rang down to the operating theatre to inform the staff. When the day of my operation arrived I decided not to have a pre-med in order to be alert for as long as possible. Arriving at the theatre, I asked the sister to check his notes. "I just want to make sure you have the correct breast down," I said, jokingly. He looked down at his notes and said, "Yes, it's the left one." I just could not believe it! To make matters worse, although the surgeon had drawn markings on the correct breast the previous day, they had washed off in the bath. I thus surrendered to the general anaesthetic, wondering whether I would wake up without the left breast, the right one or without both.

Fortunately, the correct breast was removed but, back home, it affected me for quite a while. It played on my nerves and I kept wondering what would have happened if I had taken the pre-med and not checked. Eventually, I was so stressed I asked the breast care nurse to come and talk to me. She assured me that the surgeon always works from his own notes and they were correct. It turned out to have been a clerical error. The secretary had typed 'L' instead of 'R' and every department had received a copy of her notes. I did not pursue it any further. I just wanted to forget it then and get on with my life.

I was in hospital for 17 days as I developed an infection in the wound. After a few weeks back at home, I became very depressed. For a full day I could not stop crying. Eventually I went to my GP. He is extremely compassionate. He never makes me feel that I have to rush and he always greets me by my first name. He visited me at home later that week so he could spend longer with me and he put me in touch with a local counselling group which proved to be my lifeline.

All the time I was in hospital Paul, my husband, declined all my offers to show him my scar. The day I came home I was very tired and went to bed early. I decided that, if Paul did not look at my scar that night, he never would. I thus pretended to have difficulty in getting undressed and called for him to help. That was the first time he saw the scar. Without a word he went back downstairs and did not return until 3.00am. I thought he was never going to sleep with me again! When he eventually did come to bed, he hugged me tightly and we made love. It was his way of telling me that everything would be fine.

One thing that does upset me, however, is that from the moment Paul knew I had breast cancer he stopped touching that breast. He always used to fall asleep with his hand on my right breast. He called it his dummy. In fact, when we told Paul's mother (who was 78 at the time) about my cancer, her response had been: "Well, I told you not to let our Paul fondle your breasts." As soon as he found out that I had breast cancer Paul stopped touching me there, even before the mastectomy. He explained to me that he was afraid something would come out of my breast and grab him. He just could not come to terms with the fact that there was something growing inside me. He has never touched that side since and, after 32 years of marriage, I really miss that contact.

After the operation, my arm movement did not return to normal. Twice a week for one year I had physiotherapy but there was little movement. I still could not lift it. I used to be a lorry driver, having learned that trade during a brief spell in the army. Now I was unable to load and unload so I was registered disabled.

I decided to join a Workers' Education Association evening class in local history and, helping with a W.E.A. exhibition one day, I met the Disability Access to Resources in Technology (DART) tutors. That chance meeting was to change my whole life.

I was invited to join one of their computer classes. Me! I had never touched a computer! I was far too old! I had never received much education, having left school at 15 with no 'O' levels. I was not disabled enough. The tutors must have been very persuasive because, in spite of all my protests, I found myself enrolling on a six month full-time course. After a month I was hooked. Computers were my life. I completed the course, gained my RSA certificate and was invited to stay on as a tutor. Since then, I have been on numerous courses and am now obsessed with learning. If I had not had breast cancer I would still be lorry-driving. I never thought I had any brains, only brawn! In the past, whenever I got an application form, I was unable to write anything in the section about qualifications. I can now fill it in. I know the true meaning of the saying 'Nothing lost, nothing gained'. I may have lost a breast but, by God, I have gained so much more.

Two years after my mastectomy, I saw an article about a sponsored abseil down the wall of my hospital - a 200ft drop! The words 'In aid of Cancer Research' seemed to stare at me from the page and I really felt I had no choice in the matter. I had to do it. The wall was so boring! It was concrete and the only things of interest to focus on were the cracks. I remember wishing there had been a mural painted on it. Suddenly, my left hand which was holding the rope began to burn in spite of the thick gloves I was wearing. I had been told that, if this were to happen, it would be quite safe to let go of the rope. I let go and suddenly found myself horizontal, feet against the wall, head in mid air! Then I started spinning round. Suddenly a voice from nowhere called to me, "Don't worry, Pamela. Just carry on coming down as you are." If it had not been a female voice, I would have sworn it was God talking to me. It turned out to be a woman standing far below me. I got my certificate and sweatshirt, but never again!

My legs were like jelly for five hours afterwards. I might consider a parachute jump, though!

Breast cancer has certainly changed my life - and for the better. I cannot believe the things I have done since my operation. If I die tomorrow I will not regret the opportunities I could have taken and did not.

ELEVEN STEPS TO OVERCOMING BREAST CANCER

Anon

I was forty-nine years old when breast cancer was diagnosed in 1987. I had already had a lumpectomy. I felt devastated and went quite numb. "Well, I suppose I have as much right as the next person to have breast cancer," I heard myself mutter to the surgeon who had just given me the news.

I cried all the way home and throughout the night, thinking of how my death would affect the rest of my family. How would my younger son cope with losing his Mum during his final year at University? These negative feelings lasted for about twenty-four hours and then I told myself, "You go into hospital to be cured, not to die." From that moment on I managed to think more positively most of the time. I shed a few tears after my mastectomy but then concentrated on getting my life back to normal as soon as possible. I was lucky in that I did not require any further treatment and, ten years on, I am still going strong!

Looking back, I learned a number of things which I hope will give encouragement to others facing breast cancer.

1. Remember, you are not alone. One in every twelve women develops breast cancer.
2. Think of the thousands of women who have been cured.
3. Have faith in your own treatment.
4. Keep away from 'miserable' people (those with endless sad stories).
5. Talk about your feelings, don't 'bottle-up'.
6. Have a good laugh/cry.
7. Put yourself in other people's shoes - see how they see you. Help THEM over their possible embarrassment, reassure THEM.
8. Keep busy!
9. Take inspiration from others.
10. Count all the good things in your life - make a list, including family and friends.
11. Most importantly - THINK POSITIVE! YOU CAN BEAT IT!

AFTERWORD

by

EMMELINE SMITH (Aged 10)

Hello! I am Emmeline and I am ten years old. I have a younger brother, Joshua, and a white rabbit called Tosca. I like to do drama, synchronised swimming and trampolining and I also play in a girls football team at school.

I was quite upset when my mum went into hospital to have the operation but when she came out I was glad she had done it. I think the surgeon did an excellent job. Now I am happy because I know she will not get breast cancer and we can carry on with our lives.

I know that I have a 50/50 chance of getting breast cancer. When I am older I think I would like to have the gene test because it will show if I will be at risk from breast cancer or not. If I do have the gene I will see what sort of treatment is available then.

I think it is very important to give money to help people who have got breast cancer because it will save lives.

Emmeline

COLLAGEN AND BREAST RECONSTRUCTION

Collagen are leaders in breast reconstruction implants and are very pleased to sponsor this booklet. The stories told in it give encouragement to breast cancer sufferers and we are proud that our products enable women across the world to resume their lives with real personal confidence following breast surgery. Vanessa Smith is one of these women and she has stated publicly how delighted she is with her Collagen Trilucent implants.

Breast reconstruction using implants can restore the natural shape of the breasts following mastectomies - whether done at the time of the operation or even many years later. Research with patients suggests that this reconstructive surgery has a positive influence on their healing process and self esteem.

At Collagen we are especially proud of our revolutionary Trilucent implants because of the major advantages they give women over and above conventional silicone and saline breast implants. These include:-

- Trilucent implants contain a naturally occurring vegetable oil which the body absorbs in the unlikely event of leakage, this itself being minimised by the special design and lubricating properties of the implants.
- X-Rays can pass through Trilucent implants whereas conventional saline or silicone implants can conceal between 22% and 85% of breast tissue from diagnosis.
- Safe, strong durable design, with specially textured shell to reduce scar tissue formation and subsequent breast discomfort.
- Unique protection plan and product warranty, underpinned by tiny microchips within implants, to optimise patient care.

We wish the Genesis campaign every success in identifying the causes of and cure for genetic breast cancer.

Collagen (UK) Ltd

Trilucent is a Trademark of the Collagen Corporation.

RE-ORDER FORM

To order more copies of this booklet (at £3.00 per copy, inclusive of postage and packing), please complete this form:-

Please send .... copy/copies of the booklet 'One in Twelve' to:

Name: ....

Address: ....

....Postcode...........................

Daytime Telephone Number: ....

I enclose a cheque/postal order for £..................

Please make all cheques/postal orders payable to 'The Genesis Appeal' and send to the address at the foot of this page.

DONATION FORM

I enclose a donation of £ .... to the Genesis Appeal.

Name: ....

Address: ....

....Postcode...........................

Please make all cheques/postal orders payable to 'The Genesis Appeal' and send to the address at the foot of this page.

The Genesis Appeal
The Nightingale Centre,
South Manchester University Hospitals, Nell Lane,
Manchester M20 0PT

Telephone: 0161 861 0000